ADAM DOBRZYŃSKI

SHŌTŌKAN KATAS VOL. 1
HEIAN SHODAN IN DÀOIST EYES

Adam's Shotokan Karate Books

Published in the United States
by Adam Dobrzynski at Emerald Law Group, 280 N Oak St, Ukiah, CA 95482
e-mail: adamd@mscc.huji.ac.il

Demonstration: Sophie Le Bas, Yodan, France Shōtōkan
Photography: Patrick Schoeffer, Godan, France Shōtōkan
Ken Osborne's photo: Suisse Shōtōkan Karate
Cover design: Avi Mazor
Logo design: Haya Strauss

Shotokan Katas vol. 1: Heian Shodan in Daoist Eyes
ISBN PDF: 978-1-7363447-0-5
ISBN Paperback: 978-1-7363447-1-2

For donations to the project:
Venmo: @Edie-Lerman | Pay-Pal: www.paypal.me/karatebooks

First Edition 2021

Library of Congress Cataloging-in-Publication Data
Dobrzynski, Adam.
Shotokan Katas vol. 1: Heian Shodan in Daoist Eyes / Adam Dobrzynski.
p. cm. - (martial arts)
Includes Bibliographical References and Index
ISBN: 978-1-7363447-0-5
Library of Congress Control Number: 2020926027

Dedicated to Sophie Le Bas, a warrior among warriors

SPECIAL THANKS

Editte Lerman, Esq.	Virgil McClain
Ken Osborne	Marc Zerhat
Steve Anchell	Didier Cohen
Sophie Le Bas	Freddy Finkelstein
Patrick Schoeffer	Amir Levi
Yulek Dobrzyński	Efi Greenbaum
Haya Strauss	Einav Ginesin
Yann Alezrah	Avi Mazor
Amir Shalev	Iris Akerman
Orlando Chambers	Noah Peleg
Gilles Brunot	Shimon Firman
Shalom Neaman	Lidor Blazer
Yossi Sagi	Hila Michaelson Fichtelberg
Maurício Santos	Emerald Law Group (CA)

FOREWORD

I have been asked to write a foreword for the series of books by Adam Dobrzynski. I usually decline, as there are so many others who have dedicated their lives to Budo at a higher level of understanding than myself.

Sensei Adam Dobrzynski has attained that higher level. I can say this after more than sixty years of training. This well-written, informational book is filled with treasures that will help you along your journey in martial arts. Each of us has undiscovered hidden treasures within, that have yet to be revealed.

Adam's book is full of such gems that will become yours. They will be the ones that define you and make you special. No one else will have these, only you. This book opens the door to understanding.

Ken Osborne

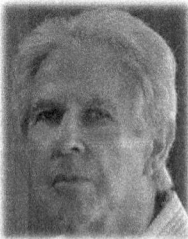

ABOUT THE FOREWORD WRITER

Shihan Ken Osborne (born 1941), is a distinguished American pioneer of Karate. Participated in the very first group of Chuck Norris. Osborne was the first to receive Norrise's black belt (1964), and the two became close partners and friends. Learning Tang Soo Do from Norris, and studying the basic athletics of Karate, made Osborne one of the strongest Kumite artists in the world. Won countless tournaments, both as a competitor and as an instructor at several Dojos. Attended the 1965 summer special training of Southern California Karate Association (SCKA), which was held at Lake Arrowhead. On his return from the famous United States Karate Congress Martial Arts Tour of Japan in 1967, Osborne joined the SCKA. Attained SKA's (Shotokan Karate of America) highest rank in record seventeen years within the organization (1984, Paris, France). Presently a member of Mumon Karate's Board of Directors, and a member of American Budō Consortium's (ABC) Board of Directors. Osborne still instructs and teaches in classes, clinics and seminars, as well as on campuses.

PRESENTATION

This is the first book in a series, which is intented to examine the links between Shotokan Karate and the three teachings – Daoism, Confucianism and Buddhism. The book deals with Heian Shodan (aka Pinan Shodan) and the rest of the Heian Katas. We can learn a lot from the Chinese origins of Karate. Daoism (Taoism) in particular has been forgotten in modern times, as a tool for understanding Karate and improving it. There are very practical conclusions that we can come to, using Daoism. In order to achieve that, we must develop a deep understanding of the Heian family using Chinese philosophy. The book explains how Yin and Yang and the Five Elements (Wuxing) theories are connected to the Heians. We especially concentrate on the Wood Element, which is the element of Heian Shodan, and which has profound implications on the Kata. Topics from Traditional Chinese Medicine (TCM) are brought up, including the relations between the basic Katas and the organs and meridians. Then we turn to Emotional Karate, and observe the psychological benefit, that one could derive from our martial art. Karate can contribute to our mental well-being. And our state of mind, as proven, affects our body - including chronic pains. After understanding the distinguishing qualities of Heian Shodan, we can understand why it is a particularly good Kata for releasing a repressed anger. As for other issues: Some techniques are presented, in order to improve the Kata and our benefit from it. We also learn how other

Katas may recuperate Heian Shodan. A mathematical formula of the five Heians is suggested, with an application to Heian Shodan's movements. Other Shotokan Katas are also mentioned – as well as specific Karate moves and stances. Finally, we warn about excessiveness, and explain how to prevent it. By the way, several interesting topics are discussed: the far and the relatively modern history of Karate and of other martial arts, our Karate ancestors and even Chinese and Japanese characters and words. In conclusion, although the book deals with Chines philosophy, it has many very applicable sides.

APOLOGY

I would like to apologize for the poor English in the book. Being a foreigner, I have tried very hard to make as little mistakes as possible, but I have no doubt that the book is still full of those. Being also destitute, I had no money to hire a linguistic editor.

I would appreciate very much any corrections You send me, for the next editions.

I intend to publish more books about Shōtōkan Karate. If any native English speaker wishes to volunteer to correct parts (not too big) of a future book, it would be greatly appreciated.

Adam Dobrzynski

adam.dob@mail.huji.ac.il

Contents

List of Figures

Chinese Roots of the Heians

§1. This book deals with Heian Shodan, the first of the Heian series. The Heians - or Pinans (or Channans) as they were called in Okinawa - can be found in Shuri-te and its successor styles, like Shōtōkan. In some classes, the Kata we call Heian Shodan is still[1] referred to as the second among the five – hence called Heian Nidan. The techniques found in the Heians, seem to come from China. More importantly, the ideas behind the techniques are Chinese. Some say that Ankō Itosu developed the Heians from Kankū-dai[2] (also called Kūsankū or Kūshankū) Kata; while others say, that Itosu assembled the Heians from Chiang Nan (Channan in Japanese approximation) Kata – both having Chinese origins. Naturally, many scholars say that the Heians are based on both Kankū and Channan[3], and perhaps on other sources. Some believe that it was Matsumura (松村), who has created the Heians from Chinese forms[4]. Few even say, that Matsumura learned a Chinese Kata named Ping An, developed one Kata out of it and called it

---

[1] Andy Pruim "A Compendium of Traditional Karate Kata: Their Origin, History and Caracteristics" 30(6) **Black Belt** 48, 49 (1992).

[2] Robin L. Rielly **Complete Shotokan Karate: The Samurai Legacy and Modern Practice** (1998) 150-151.

[3] Mark Edward Cody **Wado Ryu Karate/Jujutsu** (2008) 10.

[4] Stefano Di Marino & Roberto Ghetto **A Complete Guide to Karate** (2018) 103-104.

Pinan – that would be our Heian Shodan, also called Heian Ichi or Pinan Sono Ichi.

§2. According to one man's theory, the truth may be different. Terence Dukes (aka Nagaboshi Tomio, 1946 - 2005) claimed that since the early days of the Buddhist martial arts, the practitioner's path was designed and observed using five elements – whether they were the Hindu Mahābhūta (Pancha Maha-Bhoota) or the Chinese *wŭxíng*[5]. That was especially true for fresh disciples. Forms have been created for that purpose. In Hindu, the forms were called Mahābhūta Naṭā. Naṭā is a long sequence of movements[6], while Pratimā would be a shorter sequence[7]. Five Pratimā of the Mahābhūta Naṭā existed in China for hundreds of years before the seventh century, but around that century the Chinese began calling them *píng'ān*[8]. We have not found any sources that would support Dukes' claims about the usage of five elements in the distant past training, and about the development of forms for that aim. *Píng'ān* - sometimes transliterated as Ping An

---

[5] Nagaboshi, note 8, at p.251.

[6] Nagaboshi, note 8, at p. 490. Chris Crudelli **The Way of the Warrior: Martial Arts and Fighting Styles from Around the World** (2008) 38.

[7] Nagaboshi, note 8, at p. 220-221.

[8] Nagaboshi Tomio **The Bodhisattva Warriors: The Origin, Inner Philosophy, History and Symbolism of the Buddhist Martial Art within India and China** (2000) 252.

- means safe and sound[9], just like our Heian, and is written the same way (平安). There is a very famous Chinese insurance and finance company, called Ping An. In Korean, the Heian Katas are called Pyong Ahn and other similar names[10]; that is the same Pyong as in Pyongyang – the capital of North Korea. Pinan was the Okinawan simplified pronunciation of *píng'ān*.

§3. However, even if Itosu was the inventor of the Heians: The man was very familiar with Chinese classics[11]. Hence, if we want to delve into the Heians, we must go to their roots – the Chinese thought. That is true not only for the Heians: Historians believe that Karate was strongly influenced by Chinese fighting arts[12]. Some of our own Karate-ancestors, like Itosu[13], say that or even more. Even the non-Chinese techniques of Karate, can be related to China, since the philosophy behind them was strongly

---

[9] Clifford H. Phillips **China Beckons: An Insight to the Culture and the National Language** (1993) 251. Allen S.C. Choi **Chinese Language** (2005) 177.

[10] Udo Moenig **Taekwondo: From a Martial Art to a Martial Sport** (2015) 218.

[11] Andy Chellew **The Pinan Katas Of Shukokai and Shito-Ryu Karate: an Illustrated Guide** (2016) 2.

[12] Robin L. Rielly **Complete Shotokan Karate: History, Philosophy, and Practice** (1985) 32.

[13] Mark D. Bishop **Okinawan Karate (Kobudo & Te): Teachers, Styles and Secret Techniques** (3rd ed., 2017) 183.

influenced by Chinese ideas. Unfortunately, Karate has forgotten many of its crucial Chinese origins, especially those that came from Daoism. Some of the foundations are important for useful reasons, and not merely philosophical.

Yin, Yang and Five Phases

Fivefold Theory for Five Katas

§4.   We will do our best, to analyze Heian Shodan – as well as other Heians - using Chinese tools. The Chinese philosophy offers us several ways to understand the world, each based on a number. One of the well-known ways is established on the Two[14], dividing the world into *yīn* (Japanese: In) and *yáng* (Japanese: Yō) [15]. According to the Daoist way of thinking, the fact that there are five Heians, tells us of their character. Furthermore, the best way to analyze the Heians, would involve a fivefold theory. That is true, whether or not the Heians were intentionally planned as a system of five, and if so – why were they planned as five. It does not matter how the modern Heians came to the world, and what was the aim. Yet, we have little doubt that the Heians were indeed designed according to the *wŭxíng*. The *wŭxíng* theory of Five Elements is a fundamental part of Chinese philosophy[16]. It is a cosmological and alchemic theory, but one that has profound implications in practical fields. Those include statesmanship, economy, architecture and decoration, health, and of course –

---

[14]道德经, 二 (*Dàodé Jīng*, 2).

[15]道德经, 四十二 (*Dàodé Jīng*, 42).

[16] Zhongxian Wu **Vital Breath of the Dao: Chinese Shamanic Tiger Qigong - Laohu Gong** (2008) 60.

martial arts. In Karate, we have a lot to gain from understanding the *wŭxíng* and from implying it. The elementary Katas are a fine place to start. In our opinion, the five Heians are representatives of the Five Elements. Each Heian is based on an Element, and bears its unique properties - its own pattern or principle or laws (理 - *li*[17]).

The Elements of the Heians

§5. *Wŭxíng* (五行, sometimes transliterated as Wŭ-Hsing) can be translated as Five Elements, Five Phases, Five Processes, Five Forces, Five Activities or Five Energies. In Chinese, there are several words transliterated as *xíng*, thus we should not confuse between 行 (meaning behavior or conduct, for instance[18]) – that is the *xíng* of *wŭxíng*, 形 (meaning form or shape, for instance) and 型 (meaning type, pattern or model, for instance, and also Kata)[19]. The Five Elements are Wood, Fire, Earth, Metal and Water. Wood's direction is outwards (expansion), Fire's direction is upwards, Earth's direction is stability, Metal's direction is inwards (contraction), and Water's direction is downwards. Wood is

---

[17] **Zhu Xi: Selected Writings** (Philip J. Ivanhoe ed., 2019) 6-8.

[18] Douglas Robinson **The Deep Ecology of Rhetoric in Mencius and Aristotle: A Somatic Guide** (2016) 266.

[19] Li Dong **Tuttle Learner's Chinese-English Dictionary** (2nd ad., 2015) 201-202.

related to beginnings[20], and the Five Elements' flow traditionally starts with Wood[21], although that is not the cosmological order[22]. No wonder then, that Heian Shodan - the first Kata in many Karate disciplines - is of a Wood type. As we have said, Wood is also about spread[23], i.e. growth in all directions. The climate of Wood is wind[24], and its planet is Jupiter[25] – the biggest planet in the Solar System. In Chinese, Wood (*mù*) is written 木, and big (*dà*) is written 大. Heian Shodan is a wide Kata – its movements are long.

---

[20] Keekok Lee **The Philosophical Foundations of Classical Chinese Medicine: Philosophy, Methodology, Science** (2017) 182.

[21] Peter Acker **Liu Chuxuan 1147-1203 and His Commentary on the Daoist Scripture *Huangdi Yinfu Jing*** (2006) 23. Anita Alexandra **Elemental Art Meditation Cards: Living The Five Elements** (2009) 9.

[22] Colin A. Ronan **The Shorter Science and Civilisation in China 1** (1978) 151. Yang Li **Book of Changes and Traditional Chinese Medicine** (1998) 297. Giovanni Maciocia **The Foundations of Chinese Medicine: A Comprehensive Text** (3rd ed., 2015) 23.

[23] Gilles Marin **Five Elements, Six Conditions: A Taoist Approach to Emotional Healing, Psychology, and Internal Alchemy** (2006) 37.

[24] 素問, 五(*Sùwèn*, 5). Fabrizio Pregadio **Awakening to Reality: The "Regulated Verses" of the Wuzhen pian, a Taoist Classic of Internal Alchemy** (2009) 11.

[25] Randall L. Nadeau **The Wiley-Blackwell Companion to Chinese Religions** (2012) 54.

Heian Shodan is more Zenkutsu-dachi oriented, than any other Heian. One passes a lot of distance performing it.

§6. Heian Nidan is the Fire Kata. Fire's direction of movement is upwards. The physical fire is lighter than air – that is why it goes up. Heian Nidan begins with both hands high in the air. Fire has a rapid - even explosive - character[26], like tongues of flame. Naturally, the first opponent of Heian Nidan is dealt with bursting motions. Heian Sandan is the Earth Kata. Earth's direction of movement is center, meaning stability. Confronting the first opponent of Heian Sandan, we perform two movements (movements 2 – 3) in the same stance. And not just any stance, but a Heisoku-dachi, which demands a lot of stability. In motions 2 – 3, the hands draw a circle in front of our stomach – a classic Earth move (Figure 1 - sandan move 2, p. 48). Heian Yodan (aka Heian Yondan, Heian Shidan or Pinan Shidan) is the Metal Kata (paragraph §24). Metal's direction of movement is inwards[27]. In the first direction, we perform a movement that is slow, very precise, with sword-like open hands and with a feeling of pulling towards ourselves (Figure 12 - yodan move 1, p. 49). Those

---

[26] Bruce Frantzis **The Power of Internal Martial Arts and Chi: Combat and Energy Secrets of Ba Gua, Tai Chi and Hsing-I** (2007) 189.

[27] David Twicken **Classical Five Element Chinese Astrology Made Easy** (2000) 92.

properties are all connected to Metal. Heian Godan is the Water Kata. Water's direction of motion is downwards. That is one of the reasons to interpret the first direction, as pulling the rival down. You block his right hand attack, grab his right hand and pull it with a left Hikite - hitting him at the same time with your right hand, and then drag the opponent down slowly – putting him in front of your belly or lower (Figure 2 - godan pulling down, p. 48). The difference between Water and Earth, for example, can be seen by comparing the first movement of Heian Godan with the first movement of Heian Sandan. Performing the first move of Heian Godan, we already think about the second movement. The Ude-uke (Uchi-uke) opening Heian Sandan is more stable and decisive, but on the other side more stuck.

The Yīness and Yángness of the Heians

§7. We next turn our attention to a comparison between the language of *wǔxíng* and the language of *yīnyáng* (trad. 陰陽, simp 阴阳). In a fourfold system[28], spring or east - for instance - are *yáng* rising from *yīn*, i.e. *yáng* in *yīn* (陰中之陽). Summer or south are *yáng* in *yáng* (陽中之陽) – also called utmost *yáng*. Autumn or west are *yīn* in *yáng* (陽中之陰). And winter or north

---

[28] Paul U. Unschuld **Huang Di nei jing su wen: Nature, Knowledge, Imagery in an Ancient Chinese Medical Text** (2003) 89.

are *yīn* in *yīn* (陰中之陰[29]). In a fivefold world, Wood is *yáng* in *yīn*, Fire is *yáng* in *yáng*, Metal is *yīn* in *yáng*, and Water is *yīn* in *yīn*. That means Wood is parallel to east, for example. Earth, according to one approach, has a balance between *yáng* of *yīn* and *yīn* of *yáng*, and between *yáng* of *yáng* and *yīn* of *yīn*. It is located in the center of the compass rose[30] (Figure 3 - compass rose, p. 48). According to another approach, Earth is the extreme or ultimate *yīn* in *yīn*[31] (陰中之至陰). One can think of it, as a necessary radical intermediate-stage between the extremeness of Fire and Metal. We prefer the first approach. In a binary system – where something can be either *yīn* or *yáng*, Wood and Fire (or east and south[32]) are considered *yáng*, while Metal and Water are *yīn*. In a threefold system (next to reference 77), Earth has equal amount of *yáng* and *yīn* by one approach[33], and ultimate *yīn* by

---

[29]素問, 四 (*Sùwèn*, 4).

[30] Li Feng **Early China: A Social and Cultural History** (2013) 305-306. Robert K. Wen **Philosophy: One Man's Overview** (2014) 142.

[31]素問, 四 (*Sùwèn*, 4). 靈樞, 一 (*Lingshū*, 1). Unschuld, note 28, at p. 90-91. Chen Ming , Paul F. Ryan & Zhou Gang **Chinese Medical Classics: Selected Readings** (2014) 46. Richard Bertschinger **Essential Texts in Chinese Medicine: The Single Idea in the Mind of the Yellow Emperor** (2015) 95.

[32] Maciocia, note 22, at p. 5.

[33] Keekok Lee **The Philosophical Foundations of Classical Chinese**

another. Kiba-dachi (Figure 4 - sandan kibadachi, p. 48), which is common in Heian Sandan, can also be interpreted in both ways: From one point of view, Kiba-dachi is a middle stance, between Zenkutsu-dachi and Kōkutsu-dachi. From a second point of view, Kiba-dachi is more *yīn* than Kōkutsu-dachi. By this approach, Heian Sandan is the *yīn*iest Kata of its family.

§8. The number of slow movements in each Heian Kata is a good indication of its relative *yīn*ness or *yáng*ness. Heian Shodan and Heian Nidan, belonging to the *yáng* Elements (Wood and Fire), have zero slow movements. Heian Sandan, the Earth Kata, has one or two – depending on the version. Heian Yodan and Heian Godan, belonging to the *yīn* Elements (Metal and Water), have four and three, respectively. The ratio between Zenkutsu-dachi and Kōkutsu-dachi is also a good indication. Shodan and Nidan have more front stances than back stances. Heian Sandan has three stances of Zenkutsu and three stances of Kōkutsu. According to the first approach – the one that sees Earth as an equilibrium, Heian Sandan is between the two first Heians – which are *yáng,* and the two last Heians – which are *yīn.* The last two Heians have less Zenkutsu-dachi than Kōkutsu-dachi. The fact that Zenkutsu-dachi is generally considered *yáng*, does not mean that there is no *yīn* in it. In some aspects, such as the height, it may be more *yīn* than Kōkutsu-dachi. Some last words about the

---

Medicine: Philosophy, Methodology, Science (2017) 172-173.

dual system: In Daoism, the standard position is standing facing south[34]. Meaning that in the Yōi position (Hachiji-dachi, Shizentai, Heikō-dachi) before the Kata begins, we are presumed to face the south. Since the east is *yáng*, the fact that we begin every Heian by turning left, indicates that the Heian family consists of *yáng* Katas (paragraph §22). Heian Shodan is Wood in *yáng*, Heian Nidan is Fire in *yáng*, and so on. In the Tekkis, for instance, we go right.

---

[34] 素問, 六 (*Sùwèn*, 6). Compare: 道德经, 四十二 (*Dàodé Jīng*, 42) ("萬物負陰而抱陽").

Emotional Karate

§9. A recent study - which in fact included Heian Shodan - shows that Karate may improve emotional state[35]. We have no doubt, that the psychological benefit from training can be enhanced even further. While practicing Karate, we think much more than we feel. That way, we miss a lot of what Karate has to offer. Performing Karate, one ought to be emotionally invested. The Chinese say that stagnation of emotions – especially unexpressed Anger[36] - can stagnate the *qì*, since emotions are *qì* movements[37]. The Liver *qì* is particularly prone to stagnation resulting from repressed sentiments. The Liver is a Woody organ (next to reference 65), and so is the Gallbladder. Adding a psychological activity to our Karate movements is a much better way to use Karate for our well-being. The Five Phases Theory has a lot to contribute. According to Daoism, Wood is emotionally related to Anger[38], Fire to Hate (or Excessive Joy), Earth to

---

[35] Petra Jansen, Katharina Dahmen-Zimmer, Brigitte M. Kudielka & Anja Schulz " Effects of Karate Training Versus Mindfulness Training on Emotional Well-Being and Cognitive Performance in Later Life" 39(10) **Research on Aging** 1118, 1123, 1138 (2017).

[36] Deadman, note 124, at p. 478.

[37] Nigel Ching **The Fundamentals of Acupuncture** (2017) 168.

[38] 素問, 五(*Sùwèn*, 5). Sandra K. Anderson **The Practice of Shiatsu** (2008) 184.

Anxiety[39], Metal to Grief, and Water to Fear[40]. Since Wood is related to Anger, Heian Shodan is a perfect tool for those of us, who suffer from repressed anger; perhaps all of us do. Many – not only in the East - believe that unreleased rage influences our body as well as our sole. Even very "physical" illnesses such as back problems, are associated with stagnated anger[41]. In Chinese Medicine, fury is related to the Liver and the Gallbladder[42] - the organs themselves as well as their meridians. That idea can be compared to yellow bile (ξανθη χολή - xanthe chole) in Humorism[43]. The liver is the only visceral organ that can regenerate its tissues. Actually, a quarter of the organ could be sufficient to gain back a full liver. Like the liver, wrath has a quality of growing. Wrath grows rapidly – we may get extremely aggravated in a matter of seconds. One's anger tends to affect other people, probably more than any other emotion; it spreads well and fast. One more example, of the connection between anger and the liver, and of their qualities: When the liver is under

---

[39] Kohn, note 88, at p. 77.

[40] Lillian Bridges **Face Reading in Chinese Medicine** (2nd ed., 2012) 80.

[41] Zachary Shore **Blunder: Why Smart People Make Bad Decisions** (2008) 53 - 54.

[42] Tom Monte **The Complete Guide to Natural Healing** (1997) 525.

[43] **Webster's New World Medical Dictionary** (3rd ed., 2008) 204.

chemical stress – e.g. under the influence of alcohol – anger can rise easily. Indeed, when drunk, some of us are quick to be mad, and all of us are slow to react.

§10. It is best to practice Heian Shodan with angry eyes. In *qìgōng*, we find a technique called Punching with Angry Gaze[44] (or Punching with Fierce Eyes). This exercise is considered beneficial for the Liver, and effective in releasing bad[45] Anger[46]. The Chinese say that the Liver opens into the eyes[47] (肝氣通於目). One can understand the connection between the liver and the eyes, by thinking of yellow eyes as a very clear reflection of a troubled liver[48]. The eyes are a mediator between

---

[44] Ken Cohen "The Way of Taoist Yoga: Qigong" May/June 1997 **Yoga Journal** 95, 101.

[45] Mimi Kuo-Deemer **Qigong and the Tai Chi Axis: Nourishing Practices for Body, Mind and Spirit** (2018) 58.

[46] Scott Shetler **Abundant Health: Fitness for the Mind, Body, and Spirit** (2012) 37.

[47]靈樞, 十七 (*Lingshū*, 17). Claude Larre, Jean Schatz & Elisabeth Rochat de laVallée **Survey of Traditional Chinese Medicine** (1986) 194. Zhi Gang Sha **Soul Healing Miracles: Ancient and New Sacred Wisdom, Knowledge, and Practical Techniques for Healing the Spiritual, Mental, Emotional, and Physical Bodies** (2013) 28.

[48] JoAnn Scurlock & Burton R. Andersen **Diagnoses in Assyrian and Babylonian Medicine: Ancient Sources, Translations, and Modern Medical Analyses** (2005) 140.

the Liver and the universe[49]. Thus, the angry look is an excellent tool to release fury, especially while performing a Wood Kata like Heian Shodan. This allows us to arrive at the first important practical conclusion: While performing Heian Shodan, we want to feel angry and to look angry – particularly in our eyes.

§11. If you have started to practice Anger in your Karate, changes may occur. Pay attention to any differences, even small ones, in the ability to say no, to rise against any wrongdoing done to you, or generally to express words that do not come easy. Just make sure, you do all of these in a polite manner! Another good – but not necessary - sign, is that sometimes you laugh more easily, or that you make people laugh more easily. Alternatively, maybe your spontaneous answers and statements have improved. And generally, occasionally your words and deeds simply happen to you, as of themselves (自然 - *zìrán*, 無爲 - *wú wéi*), without thinking. Wishfully, you will ask yourself from time to time "did that really come from me so naturally?"

---

[49] Wei Qi-ping, Andy Rosenfarb & Liang Li-na **Ophthalmology in Chinese Medicine** (2011) 26.

Wood Qualities

Stretching

§12. In Chinese, there is a phrase called *sōng* (松, 鬆[50]), which means loose[51]. In martial arts, *sōng* means loosening[52], not necessarily physiologically, in order to stretch out[53]. 松 also means a pine[54]. In Japanese, 松村 is Matsumura[55], Ankō Itosu's and Funakoshi's teacher, and 松濤 is Shōtō – Funakoshi's pen name. Shōtō-kan is written 松濤館. The expending-outgoing[56]

---

[50] Maosong Sun, Yang Liu & Jun Zhao **Chinese Computational Linguistics and Natural Language Processing Based on Naturally Annotated Big Data** (2016) 219.

[51] Michael Burkhardt **TPS Frequency Dictionary of Mandarin Chinese** (2010) 251.

[52] Mathew Mathews **The Singapore Ethnic Mosaic: Many Cultures, One People** (2018) 79.

[53] Andrea Falk **Falk's Dictionary of Chinese Martial Art: Chinese to English** (2019) 299.

[54] Ian Low **Chinese to English Dictionary (Traditional Characters)** (2012) 141. Shawn Arthur **Early Daoist Dietary Practices: Examining Ways to Health and Longevity** (2013) 97.

[55] Bruce D. Clayton **Shotokan's Secret: The Hidden Truth Behind Karate's Fighting Origins** (2004) 106.

[56] Neil Ripski **Secrets of Drunken Boxing 3: Internal Alchemy** (2018) 140.

energy is called *péng jìn*, 掤 being the character for *péng*. The radical 木 in the beginning of both 松 (*sōng*) and 掤[57] (*péng*) stands for wood. Performing the Woody and big Heian Shodan, we have an exceptionally good opportunity to imagine and to feel our joints expanding[58], i.e. the bones get further and further apart from each other. The shoulder, for instance, is easy to test: The spaced position, when the shoulder is 90° flexed (as in Oi-zuki), creates a sulcus just distal to the lateral edge of the acromion[59] (Figure 5 - oizuki, p. 48). Some people can easily create that dimple on their right shoulder, but find the task harder on the left side. *Sōng* does not refer solely to the joints: We should feel that whatever can be opened and lengthened in our body does indeed open and lengthen. That is a special way of relaxation, since it is active. Actually, some of our muscles – such as the chest and many of the *yáng* muscles (extensors) - work harder in the pulled-out position. Paradoxically, one of the main purposes of *sōng* is

---

[57] Jonathan Bluestein Shifu **Research of Martial Arts** (2014) 326.

[58] Davidine Siaw-Voon Sim & David Gaffney **Chen Style Taijiquan: The Source of Taiji Boxing** (2002) 153.

[59] Brian J. Cole & Jon K. Sekiya **Surgical Techniques of the Shoulder, Elbow and Knee in Sports Medicine** (2008) 98. Mark Dennis, William Talbot Bowen & Lucy Cho **Mechanisms of Clinical Signs** (2012) 48.

to gather the body into one solid unit[60]. Just like a tree in a good shape, it is neither stiff nor floppy, but can ward off (*péng*[61]) when pushed hard enough. A force put against our hand, should be transferred to the ground[62], but not harshly. Heian Shodan is not a Metal Kata; hence, the body should feel more like a rubber than a metal. One can imagine Newton's Cradle with elastic balls.

Flow

§13. By Chinese philosophy, Wood should be in constant movement[63]. It likes to move, more than any other element[64]. In TCM (Traditional Chinese Medicine), Wood is responsible for a smooth flow of *qì* and blood in the body; *qì* is pronounced Ki in Japanese - as in Kiai. The *yīn* organ of Wood is the Liver[65]

---

[60] Oleg Tcherne **Alchemy of Pushing Hands** (2009) 123.

[61] Rick Barrett **Taijiquan: Through the Western Gate** (2006) 248. Wang Shujin **Bagua Swimming Body Palms** (2011) 86.

[62] Michael W. Acton **Eternal Spring: Taijiquan, Qi Gong, and the Cultivation of Health, Happiness and Longevity** (2009) 186-187.

[63] Jason Elias & Katherine Ketcham **Chinese Medicine for Maximum Immunity: Understanding the Five Elemental Types for Health and Well-Being** (1999) 24.

[64] John Kirkwood **The Way of the Five Seasons: Living with the Five Elements for Physical, Emotional, and Spiritual Harmony** (2016) 147.

[65] 王冰, 素問, 二 (*Wáng Bīng* on *Sùwèn*, 5).

(paragraph §9), and the Gallbladder (paragraph §19) is Wood's *yáng* organ[66]. Smoothness is very important to the Liver, and it is extremely prone to stagnation[67]. Heian Shodan ought to be performed flowingly. One can practice, even sitting or lying, shortening the interval between inhalation and exhalation and vice versa, thinking of smooth transitions between the two[68]. In Heian Shodan itself, one should not pause[69] too much between the movements and between the adversaries.

§14. In one case, since it was technically possible, two movements were officially joint to one. That was the case of the second and the third motions of the third direction (movements 7–8 of Heian Shodan)[70] (Figure 6 - shodan move 7, p. 48). Interestingly, counting the two movements as one, changes the total number of movements in the five Heians from 122 to 121. Unlike the western culture, numerology in traditional China is part

---

[66] Kohn, note 88, at p. 74.

[67] Zhanwen Liu Liang Liu & **Essentials of Chinese Medicine 1** (2009) 28.

[68] Bruce Frantzis **Opening the Energy Gates of Your Body: Chi Gung for Lifelong Health** (1993) 245-246.

[69] Lawrence A. Kane & Kris Wilder **The Way of Kata: A Comprehensive Guide to Deciphering Martial Applications** (2005) 136, 141.

[70] Gichin Funakoshi **Karate-Dō Kyōhan: The Master Text** (trans. by Tsutomu Ohshima, 2012) 50 [Funakoshi 1935 Ohshima].

of the mainstream philosophy. We do not mean the auspicious-inauspicious theories – which of course have a lot of wisdom and depth as for themselves, but the substantive numerology. Understanding the number could mean grasping the very essence. If we understand why the Two and the Four both have a disintegrative quality, we may understand why Heian Nidan and Heian Yodan do not begin with a movement that involves crossing the hands - but with separation (paragraph §23) (Figure 7 - nidan separation, p. 48). The Five, by the way, has an organizing quality. Thus the Heians, by their very number, are an effort to put knowledge into order.

§15. Debatably, Heian Shodan has 21^{71} motions in its "longer" version, Heian Nidan has 26^{72}, Heian Sandan has 23^{73}, Heian Yodan has 27^{74} and Heian Godan has 25^{75} – together they add up to 122 movements. One hundred twenty-two has no significant meaning in mathematics or in the Chinese culture. One hundred twenty-one though, has a lot: 121 is a square, and not just any

---

[71] SHODAN 21: Funakoshi 1935 Ohshima, note 70, at p. 48. Gichin Funakoshi **Karate Dō Kyōhan: Master Text for the Way of the Empty-Hand** (trans. by Harumi Suzuki-Johnston, 2nd ed., 2012) 43 [Funakoshi 1935 Suzuki]. Gichin Funakoshi **To-Te Jitsu** (trans. by Shingo Ishida, 1997) 210 [Funakoshi 1925 Ishida]. Gichin Funakoshi **Karate Jutsu – the Original Teachings of Master Funakoshi** (trans. by John Teramoto, 2001) 128 [Funakoshi 1925 Teramoto]. Joachim Grupp **Shotokan Karate Kata 2** (2nd ed., 2007) 21.

[72] NIDAN 26: Funakoshi 1935 Ohshima, note 70, at p. 54. Funakoshi 1935 Suzuki, note 71, at p. 51 . Funakoshi 1925 Ishida, note 71, at p. 69. Funakoshi 1925 Teramoto, note 71, at p. 58. Grupp, note 71, at p. 21.

[73] SANDAN 23: Funakoshi 1935 Ohshima, note 70, at p. 62. Funakoshi 1935 Suzuki, note 71, at p. 57.

[74] YODAN 27: Funakoshi 1935 Ohshima, note 70, at p. 71. Funakoshi 1935 Suzuki, note 71, at p. 62. Funakoshi 1925 Ishida, note 71, at p. 220. Funakoshi 1925 Teramoto, note 71, at p. 134. Grupp, note 71, at p. 21.

[75] GODAN 25: Funakoshi 1935 Ohshima, note 70, at p. 79. Funakoshi 1935 Suzuki, note 71, at p. 67.

square, but the only one of the form $p^0+p^1+p^2+p^3+p^4$ - that is to say $1+p+p^2+p^3+p^4$, where p is prime[76]. Pay attention to the fact that $p=3$ and to the fact, that there are five terms on the left-hand side of the equation $(p^0+p^1+p^2+p^3+p^4=121)$. These are not coincidences. The Heian series is a world based on the Three (The Trinitarian Principle of Heaven, Earth, and Man[77]) and the Five (*wǔxíng*); both the Three and the Five represent unity. Maybe originally moves seven and eight of Heian Shodan were one, and only later, that single movement was separated for didactic reasons. On the other hand, there is another count in which Heian Sandan has 24[78] movements and not 23, and Heian Godan has 23[79] movements and not 25. In that case, the 21 motions of the "longer" Heian Shodan, do add up to 121 with the other Heians - therefore the "longer" count of Heian Shodan was the original. It also might be noted, that the Chinese checkers board, shaped like the Star of David, consists of 121 holes[80].

---

[76] Jean-Marie De Koninck **Those Fascinating Numbers** (2009) 39.

[77] 禮記, 九 - 禮運 (*Lǐjì, 9 - Lǐyùn*). Benebell Wen **The Tao of Craft: Fu Talismans and Casting Sigils in the Eastern Esoteric Tradition** (2016) 10 - 13.

[78] SANDAN 24: Funakoshi 1925 Ishida, note 71, at p. 215. Funakoshi 1925 Teramoto, note 71, at p. 131.

[79] GODAN 23: Funakoshi 1925 Ishida, note 71, at p. 225. Funakoshi 1925 Teramoto, note 71, at p. 137.

[80] Claudi Alsina & Roger B. Nelsen **Icons of Mathematics: An**

Heaven and Earth

§16. After the open-handed Age-uke, come three more (Figure 8 - ageuke, p. 48). Four movements in a raw, in the same "opponent" (i.e. facing the same direction), seem unique. One could think that the reason is the sequential character of Heian Shodan – and of Wood. Nevertheless, we find this phenomenon also in Taikyoku Yodan[81] (in some of its versions) and Taikyoku Rokudan basic Katas; Taikyoku in Chinese is *tàijí*, known as T'ai Chi. We find four consecutive movements facing the same direction, also in Bassai Dai and Bassai Shō (Shutō-uke), and arguably in Empi (Teishō Oshi-age-uke). We think there is a more important reason for the sequence, having to do with the movement itself rather than the continuity: Many in the world consider trees to be connectors between Heaven and Earth[82]. In *qìgōng*, we find a tree-like exercise in which one palm goes down and the other goes up, called Connecting Heaven and Earth. Connecting Heaven and Earth bears some resemblance to Age-uke, and is considered a Wood exercise.

Exploration of Twenty Key Images (2011) 210.

[81] Patrick McDermott & Ferol Arce **Karate's Supreme Ultimate: The Taikyoku Kata in Five Rings** (2004) 92.

[82] Peg Streep **Spiritual Gardening: Creating Sacred Space Outdoors** (1999) 47.

§17. We have mentioned *tàijí* (trad. 太極 ,simp. 太极), or Taikyoku in Japanese (Figure 9 - old characters for Taikyoku, p. 48). *Tàijí* is a deep and old term in Chinese cosmology[83]. It could mean the source, the beginning, the great supreme, the supreme ultimate, the great pole, the supreme polarity[84], the highest top etcetera. Personally, we think that *tàijí* is the One, not exactly the *Dào* on one side and not the Two on the other side. The One is what *Dào* gave birth to, and what created the Two[85]. According to some Chinese classics, *tàijí* generates the *yáng* and the *yīn*, and those generate the Five Elements[86]. Practicing the Taikyoku (*tàijí*) Katas, will enable us to have good Heians. We would strongly recommend practicing Taikyoku Shodan a bit, before learning Heian Shodan.

---

[83]朱子語類，理氣上 (*Zhūzi yǔ lèi, Lǐqì shàng*).

[84] Wm. Theodore De Bary & Irene Bloom **Sources of Chinese Tradition 1: From Earliest Times to 1600** (2nd ed., 1999) 673-674. Joseph A. Adler **Reconstructing the Confucian Dao: Zhu Xi's Appropriation of Zhou Dunyi** (2014) 113.

[85]道德经, 四十二 (*Dàodé Jīng*, 42).

[86] Koo Dong Yun **The Holy Spirit and Ch'i (Qi): A Chiological Approach to Pneumatology** (2012) 53. Justin Tiwald & Bryan W. Van Norden **Readings in Later Chinese Philosophy: Han Dynasty to the 20th Century** (2014) 136.

The Cycles

Strengthening Wood - The Generating Cycle

§18. The Five Phases theory states, that Wood generates Fire. That seems natural, since wood is probably the most common feed. Fire generates Earth. One way to think about it is to remember that our planet used to be all fire. Another way is to think of fire ash, which becomes earth. Earth generates Metal. Ore deposits are mined from the earth[87]. Metal generates Water. Metal in the ground might arouse rainfall[88]. Iron and minerals are absorbed into the groundwater in the aquifers[89]. Alternatively, we can think of car hoods, collecting due during the night. And Water generates Wood – plants cannot live without water. So Wood feeds Fire, Fire creates Earth, Earth bears Metal, Metal collects Water, and Water nourishes Wood[90] (Figure 10 - generating cycle,

---

[87] Pamela D. Winfield "Materializing the Zen Monastery" **Zen and Material Culture** (Pamela D. Winfield & Steven Heine ed., 2017) 37, 44.

[88] Livia Kohn **Science and the Dao – From the Big Bang to Lived Perfection** (2016) 72.

[89] Sharoz Kumar Sharma **Adsorptive Iron Removal from Groundwater (IHE Dissertation)** (2001) 4.

[90] Wu Hung **The Art of the Yellow Springs: Understanding Chinese Tombs** (2010) 152.

p. 49). In order to strengthen Wood, we have to strengthen Water. One way to improve Heian Shodan is simply to practice Heian Godan – the Water Kata. Parenthetically, since Earth supports all Elements[91], every Kata would benefit from practicing Heian Sandan; Heian Sandan teaches us to ground ourselves.

§19. Another way to improve the Kata is to add Water into Heian Shodan itself. The next two paragraphs will demonstrate, how Water could be added to the Kata directly. Heian Shodan, as previously mentioned, is an extremely Woody Kata, connected to the Gallbladder. As stated in Chinese classics, the Gallbladder is crucial for courage[92], decision-making[93] and determination. The Liver, by the way, is also important for courage[94]. The Gallbladder must function well, in order for one to make a decision to start something or to change something. The beginning of every movement in Karate requires some measure of decisiveness. Indeed, improving that mental ability to go from

---

[91] Angela Hicks, John Hicks & Peter Mole **Five Element Constitutional Acupuncture** (2nd ed., 2011) 107.

[92] Meihua Zheng **A Conceptual Metaphor Account of Word Composition: Potentiality of "Light" in English and Chinese** (2017) 79 - 90.

[93] 素問, 八(*Sùwèn*, 8). Bob Flaws & Philippe Sionneau **The Treatment of Modern Western Medical Diseases with Chinese Medicine** (2nd ed., 2005) 19.

[94] Deadman, note 124, at p. 478. Kohn, note 88, at p. 77.

stillness into swift action - or any other beginning or change, would advance every Karate movement. The Gallbladder is even more important, when starting a Kata, and most crucial in the beginning of Heian Shodan. It takes a lot of resolve to begin a Kata - namely a fight, with two big steps of Zenkutsu-dachi towards the attacker. Heian Shodan is the only Kata, besides some of the Taikyokus, which opens with a Zenkutsu-dachi towards the rival.

§20. If we want to know what the beginning of a Heian Shodan should feel like, we can have some mental exercise at home. This exercise does take practice, but can be a miracle worker. First, we take few moments to connect to ourselves. We can sit with closed eyes and concentrate on our breath, for instance, and imagine ourselves walking calmly and pleasantly in a forest. After that part of concentrating and relaxation, which is not easy at all, we shall practice Fear. If we do not feel Fear properly, we cannot continue to determination. Fear, as mentioned above, is associated with Water. Without the Water Phase, one cannot produce good Wood, since Water nourishes Wood. Hence, suddenly we see a bear at about our height. The change from calm to frightened is sudden and drastic. We run from the bear, and it chases us. One should feel the fear very vividly, and for a rather long time. We must visualize the chase, and the horror that accompanies our escape. One should try to devote himself to the fear. That is not an easy meditation. Regularly, we are somewhat detached from our feelings in general[95] and from fear especially. However, as mentioned above, without Fear we cannot develop the Wood Element, which is the element of Heian Shodan. So, we are running away from the bear. Then something changes in our hart. Maybe we suddenly realize that we cannot outrun the bear, since it has more endurance than we do, and we will only tire ourselves running. Maybe we suddenly realize that we stand a fair chance against it. Maybe we suddenly recall that running from a bear is dangerous[96]. Or maybe we just suddenly do not like the feeling of running away. We come to a rapid conclusion, that this is it, and turn around in order to confront the bear. The feeling is abrupt, very powerful, and short. That brief moment of rotating and looking at the bear, is a unique moment, with a sparkle in it. That sparkle[97] should be present in the beginning of Heian Shodan, or any Kata. This mental exercise is a very good way to bring energy from the Water Element, to strengthen Wood. At the Dōjō, feeling fear before beginning Heian Shodan, will improve the Kata as well.

---

[95] Daniel Perret **The Experience of Spirituality – A Meditation between Heaven and Earth** (2011) 13.

[96] Dave Smith **Backcountry Bear Basics: The Definitive Guide to Avoiding Unpleasant Encounters** (2nd ed., 2006) 87.

[97] Nancy Mellon & Ashley Ramsden **Body Eloquence: The Power of Myth and Story to Awaken the Body's Energies** (2008) 61.

Weakening Wood - The Controlling Cycle

§21. In the Wood Phase, there is a danger of growing too fast, growing in a bad direction and overgrowing[98]. Fresh trainees performing Heian Shodan suffer from a double risk, since they are at the Wood stage of their training, and practice a Wood Kata. If they are young in age as well, the risk is even greater. Let us take an example of the danger: We have said, that Heian Shodan should be performed smoothly (paragraph §13). Nevertheless, the Kata is liable to become too quick or too scattered. We may unintentionally cultivate too much Anger. The Liver-*qi* has that nature, of easily becoming flamed[99] (paragraph §9). One way to prevent excess Wood is to reduce Water. Another way is to put boundaries. Just like a sapling needs a stake or an iron tube, to direct its growth and to protect it. Wood-Fire-Earth-Metal-Water is named The Generating Cycle. It is also called The Creative Cycle, The Engendering Cycle, and The Mutual Production Order. There is another cycle in *wǔxíng* (五行)[100], called The Controlling

---

[98] Deadman, note 124, at p. 478.

[99] John Kirkwood **The Way of the Five Elements: 52 Weeks of Powerful Acupoints for Physical, Emotional, and Spiritual Health** (2016) 135.

[100] Gary Dolowich **Archetypal Acupuncture: Healing with the Five Elements** (2003) 66-67.

Cycle[101], The Overcoming Cycle, The Conquest Cycle, or The Destructive Cycle (Figure 11 - controlling cycle, p. 49). As per it[102], Metal overcomes Wood. The ax chops the wood. Water overcomes Fire – this we can easily understand. Wood overcomes Earth. Plants cover the ground, and pierce it while growing. Fire overcomes Metal. The fire melts the metal. And Earth overcomes Water. Banks of a river are a good example, and so are dams. If there is a lack of clarity in Heian Shodan, one should add Metal to it, since Metal controls Wood[103]. We shall explain how Metal could be added to Heian Shodan down the road (paragraphs §24-§25).

---

[101] Kiiko Matsumoto & Stephen Birch **Five Elements and Ten Stems: *Nan Ching* Theory, Diagnostics and Practice** (1983) 28.

[102]難經,七十五 (*Nán Jīng*, 75)

[103] R. Barry Harmon **Kuk Sool Goong: Korean Martial Art Archery** (2017) 50.

Shū Movements

§22. Heian Shodan is the only Heian, in which the first two rivals are not symmetrical. There is an odd number of movements in the first two directions. The fact that they contain five movements may not be incidental. Perhaps those movements are a "microcosm" of the Five Heians – and of the Five Phases. In TCM, there are so-called *shū* points[104] (*shū* means transport). *Wǔ shū* (五輸)[105] points are five acupuncture locations on our distal extremities[106], each related to an Element, arranged according to the Generating Cycle[107]. On the *yīn* meridians (such as the Liver meridian), the first point is Wood, and on the *yáng* meridians (such as the Gallbladder meridian) the five points begin with Metal[108].

---

[104] Stevenson Xutian , Tai Shusheng & Chun-Su Yuan **Handbook Of Traditional Chinese Medicine 1** (2014) 92-93.

[105] Peter C. van Kervel **Acupuncture Celestial Treatments for Terrestrial Diseases: Causes and Development of Diseases & Treatment Principles and Strategies** (2010) 186.

[106] Yu Hui-chan & Han Fu-ru **Golden Needle Wang Le-ting: A 20th Century Master's Approach to Acupuncture** (1997) 51.

[107] Hans-Ulrich Hecker, Angelika Steveling, Elmar T. Peuker & Joerg Kastner **Practice of Acupuncture: Point Location-Treatment Options-TCM Basics** (2005) 44–45.

[108] 難經, 六十四 (*Nán Jīng*, 64). Xia Fei & Mu Jianhua **Advanced TCM Series 6: Acupuncture and Moxibustion** (Chen Ping ed., 2000) 46.

By that count, assuming that Heian Shodan is a *yīn*-Wood Kata (after reference 115), its fourth step – the withdrawal back (paragraph §25), would be a Metal move (Wood-Fire-Earth-Metal). There are reasons for *yīn* Katas to begin with Wood. Firstly, it takes Wood to get the *yīn* moving. Secondly, since we open the five movements with Wood, the last movement is Water (Wood-Fire-Earth-Metal-Water). Water, disputably (next to reference 31), is the most *yīn* Element[109]. Placing the Water motion in the end of the five transport movements ensures that the rest of the Kata would continue with a *yīn* energy and remain *yīn*. In Heian Shodan's case, that would be the *yīn* aspect of Wood - which is by itself *yáng*ish[110]. To be precise, Heian Shodan is *yīn* of Wood within the *yáng*, since the Heians are *yáng* (paragraph §8). The Heian Katas tend to resemble the northern styles of Chinese martial arts. Those are more related to Shuri-te and Tomari-te (Shōrin-ryū), than to Naha-te (Shōrei-ryū). Note that Shōrin (少林) is simply *Shàolín*. Anyways, experts may take into

---

[109] Peter Mole **Acupuncture for Body, Mind and Spirit** (2014) 53. John Kirkwood **The Way of the Five Seasons: Living with the Five Elements for Physical, Emotional, and Spiritual Harmony** (2016) 87.

[110] 丁锦, 難經, 六十四 (*Dīng Jǐn* on *Nán Jīng*, 64).

account, that *Yīn*-Wood is the second of the Ten Heavenly Stems (*yǐ*)[111] and the fourth of the Twelve Earthly Branches (*mǎo*)[112].

§23. We have talked about relativity – the fact that Heian Shodan is *yīn* of Wood, but within the *yáng*. The Chinese thought process is usually less dichotomous than the Western one. When we say that the first movement of Heian Shodan is *yáng* (Wood), we present only part of the full picture. On another level, the first move is *yīn*, since it is probably a defense: The defense is followed by our attack, which would be the *yáng* between the two movements. Another example: On the one hand, Heian Nidan and Heian Yodan are very different – Nidan is *yáng* (Fire) while Yodan is *yīn* (Metal). However, from a different point of view, the second (2) and the fourth (4) Katas are very similar, belonging to the even numbers. That is why these separative Katas (paragraph §14), do not contain even a single Oi-zuki. In our opinion, Oi-zuki symbolizes unity.

---

[111] 難經, 六十四 (*Nán Jīng*, 64). Eva Wong **Harmonizing Yin and Yang: The Dragon-tiger Classic** (1997) 11.

[112] David Twicken **I Ching Acupuncture - The Balance Method: Clinical Applications of the Ba Gua and I Ching** (2012) 94.

The Tools

Adding Metal to Heian Shodan

§24. Our tools for balancing the Five Elements are found in the Kata itself as well as outside it. External fortification of Metal, in order to reduce Wood, can be done by practicing Heian Yodan - the fourth Kata. Heian Yodan has many open hands movements, acting like a sword. Sharpness, naturally, is associated with Metal[113]. Shutō-uke, for example, is so *yīn*ish, that we rarely see it performed in a Zenkutsu-dachi. The slow movements in the beginning of Heian Yodan are done with open palms. These two motions are extremely Metallic (paragraph §6). Being slow, they seem almost the opposite of the Gallbladder-determination. Metal stands for refinement and precision. However, refinement and precision do not contradict the feeling of letting go. On the contrary. The two movements ought to be performed in the easiest, simplest and shortest way, as if one has thrown off all the obstacles of his body and soul. Therefore, Heian Yodan is calm – even melancholic, and very exact. If you feel like a puppy running all over the place while performing Heian Shodan, with imprecise movements and hands thrown in the air, Heian Yodan will concentrate you. For that, among other techniques, there are no less than four Morote-ukes in Heian Yodan.

---

[113] Kohn, note 88, at p. 72.

§25. Internal fortification of Metal in Heian Shodan can be achieved, by beginning the last two Age-ukes with open front hand. Opening the fists slows the pace down, and adds calmness and order. Originally, it seems, those Age-ukes indeed used to begin by opening the front palms. The same goal can be achieved, by paying extra attention to the fourth movement of Heian Shodan. The fourth movement, being Metal (paragraph §22), is there to calm the Wood. Learning to step back is crucial for building the right character – a human character as well as a warrior's character. Fresh students of Karate need Metal in Heian Shodan, in order to learn anger-control (paragraph §21). The closing section of Heian Shodan[114] – the Shutō-ukes, has the same roll of restricting Wood (Figure 13 - shodan last move, p. 49). Those four movements are a good way to end the Wood Kata, by putting boundaries. If we may simplify, again, Kōkutsu-dachi is a *yīn* stance by nature, making it closer to Metal and Water then to Wood and Fire. The openhanded movement (Shutō-uke) adds the Metal quality[115]. The Metal in Heian Shodan may explain,

---

[114] Chris Tomas "The Evolution of Shotokan Karate: How and Why Gichin Funakoshi Forumulated His Fighting System" 27(9) **Black Belt** 30, 32 (1989).

[115] Metal and sword: Gilles Marin **Five Elements, Six Conditions: A Taoist Approach to Emotional Healing, Psychology and Internal Alchemy** (2006) 51.

why this Kata should be classified as a *yīn*-Wood (paragraph §22) – and not a *yáng*-Wood – Kata. Another method of calming Wood in Heian Shodan, is to separate movements 7 – 8 of the Kata.

The Basics of Balancing

§26. If we have too much Wood in Heian Shodan, we can also soften and quiet the first movement (Wood), and tonify the forth (Metal). The doctrine is, of course, much wider - and on the other hand tailor-made. Here are some strategies[116] in a nutshell, just for the taste of it: If we do not have enough Anger (Wood) because we lack Fear (Water), we should strengthen both. We can do that, for instance, by emphasizing the first and the fifth movements of Heian Shodan – both begin with a narrow standing. If we lack Anger (Wood) because we have too much Grief (Metal), we can "weaken" the forth move in any way – e.g. with a feeling of going forward although we withdraw. If we have an excess of Anger (Wood) because a deficiency of Grief (Metal), we can fortify the forth movement and sedate the first, as mentioned above. If the Wood has flamed, we can sedate the second movement. Sometimes the second step of Heian Shodan swallows the first – and then we have to perform the second move with ease. If we lack speed (Fire) because of a Wood deficiency, we should strengthen the second movement as well as the first.

---

[116] Chang Sok Suh **Acupuncture Anatomy: Regional Micro-Anatomy and Systemic Acupuncture Networks** (2016) 10.

The Third Movement

§27. Another physical example: If we lack smoothness (Wood) because we try very hard to be stable (Earth) during Heian Shodan, we should perform the third movement more lightly (Figure 14 - shodan move 3, p. 49). That has to do, while on the subject, with yet another cycle of *wǔxíng* - called the Insulting Cycle[117]. And vice versa: If we lack stability (Earth) because of too much Wood in Heian Shodan, we need to emphasize the turn – which is an Earth movement. The third movement of Heian Shodan is also a *yuán* (原) movement. In TCM, *yuán* (meaning original or primary) point is a location, in which we find the original *qì* of the meridian[118]. In *yīn* meridians, such as the Liver, it is the third[119] *shū* point – the Earth point[120]. Hence, the third movement of the Kata is the one that reminds us of Heian Shodan's nature. This step is exceptionally big and difficult to perform. We should emphasize the turn, and perform it very widely. Originally, all *yīn*

---

[117] Serge Augier **Ba Zi - The Four Pillars of Destiny: Understanding Character, Relationships and Potential Through Chinese Astrology** (2017) 44.

[118] Ren Zhang **World Century Compendium To Tcm 6: Introduction To Acupuncture And Moxibustion** (2013) 42.

[119] 徐大椿, 難經, 六十四 (*Xú Dàchūn* on *Nán Jīng*, 64).

[120] Andrew Ellis, Nigel Wiseman, Ken Boss & James Cleaver **Fundamentals of Chinese Acupuncture** (revised ed., 2004) 436.

yuán points' kanjis (including the Heart's[121]), used to begin with 大 (*dà* - big, great) or 太 (*tài* - highest, supreme). The Liver meridian's *yuán* point - *tàichōng* (太沖), which is parallel to Heian Shodan's third step, is translated as Supreme Surge[122], Supreme Assault[123], Great Rushing[124] and the like. *Tàichōng* (LV-3) may be the most important point on the Liver's meridian[125]. By the by, *tàichōng*, which is located on the proximal first metatarsal space, is a great target for a Fumi-komi (Figure 15 - liv-3, p. 49). We believe that the third movement is the most significant motion of Heian Shodan. It is the golden move of the Kata.

§28. There are two ways to perform the third movement of Heian Shodan - as the rest of the turns. In the Woody way, the feeling is large throughout the entire turn. The hands are used as a tail, swinging widely like tree branches. This style could be seen in Hirokazu Kanazawa's (1931 – 2019) Heian Shodan performance

---

[121] Andrew Ellis, Nigel Wiseman & Ken Boss **Grasping the Wind** (1989) 417-418.

[122] Nigel Wiseman & Feng Ye **A Practical Dictionary of Chinese Medicine** (2nd ed., 1998) 484.

[123] Yves Requena **Terrains and Pathology in Acupuncture 1: Correlations with Diathetic Medicine** (1986) 200. Georges Soulié de Morant **Chinese Acupuncture** (1994) 501.

[124] Peter Deadman, Mazin Al-Khafaji & Kevin Baker **A Manual of Acupuncture** (2001) 477-478, 635, 638.

[125] Deadman, note 124, at p. 478.

(available on YouTube). In the Metallic way, we are contracted in the middle of the turn – and only then open ourselves again to finish the move (Figure 16 - move 3 Metal style, p. 49). A scattered practitioner, with too much Wood, is advised to perform the turns – and especially Heian Shodan's third movement – the Metallic way.

Pictures

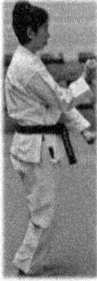

Figure 1 - sandan move 2

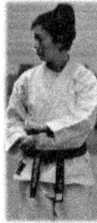

Figure 2 - godan pulling down

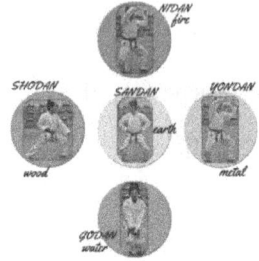

Figure 3 - compass rose

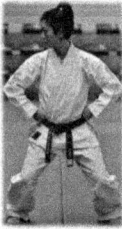

Figure 4 - sandan kibadachi

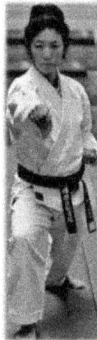

Figure 5 - oizuki

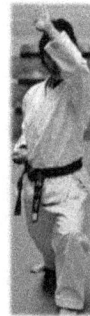

Figure 6 - shodan move 7

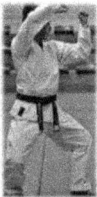

Figure 7 - nidan separation

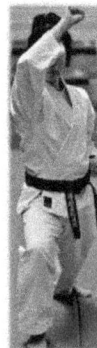

Figure 8 - ageuke

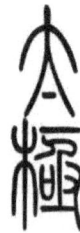

Figure 9 - old characters for Taikyoku

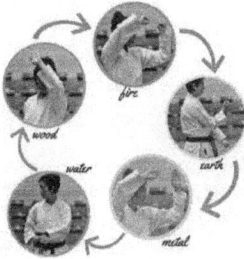

Figure 10 - generating cycle

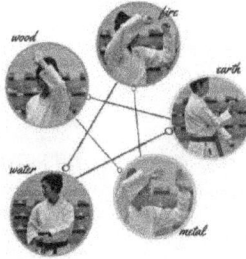

Figure 11 - controlling cycle

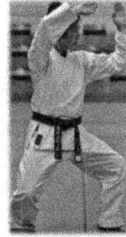

Figure 12 - yodan move 1

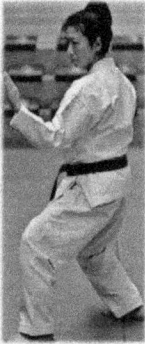

Figure 13 - shodan last move

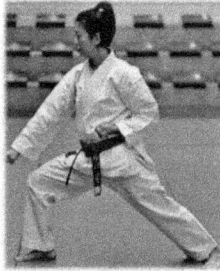

Figure 14 - shodan move 3

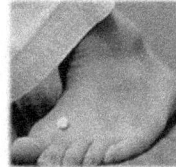

Figure 15 - liv-3

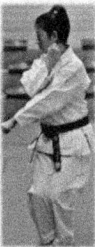

Figure 16 - move 3 Metal style

Index

www.ingramcontent.com/pod-product-compliance
Lightning Source LLC
Chambersburg PA
CBHW020438030426
42337CB00014B/1307